Herbal Remedies Secrets

You Wish You Knew

Disclaimer

Summary

Want to go au natural? Herbal remedies are 100% natural and are made using the ingredients that are easily available in Nature. Certain ingredients can also be grown at home or they can be easily found in a farmer's market near your home.

With the remedies mentioned in this eBook, you'll be able to soothe your body and your mind. Whether you want something that will help soothe your tired muscles, lift your spirits or improve your health, the recipes contained within this eBook will be useful in almost any situation.

With the help of this eBook, we'll introduce you to herbal remedies through:

- Detailed step by step instructions for various methods.

- Critical information on which recipes to use for which condition.

- Small section on how to make herbal oils, tinctures and creams.

Herbal remedies have been utilized by people for quite a long time. While some people dismiss them as old wives' tales or recipes that were believed to be effective in older times, herbal remedies are still capable of producing results.

No matter what the affliction may be, these herbal remedies are able to help ease or soothe them. Try out the recipes in this eBook and see which ones soothe you.

Contents

Introduction to Herbal Remedies

Herbal remedies have been in our history for centuries and it is possible to find herbal remedy recipes for almost any ailment. Designed in a time when there wasn't much scope in pharmaceutical medicines, many herbal remedies come from Chinese, Japanese or Indian descents. Herbal remedies also earn more preference over pharmaceutical medication owing to the fact that such medication often uses herbal extracts.

However, they're considered more harmful and have a wider array of side effects owing to the fact that they have synthetic chemicals added to them as well. On the other hand, herbal remedies were popularly utilized since their ingredients produced little to no side effects.

For people who're looking for a way to soothe their everyday aches and pains, these herbal remedies can prove to be really useful. For someone who has to resort to consuming pharmaceutical medicine for their everyday ailment meant having to deal with the side effects and fighting the addiction to that drug as well.

Going back to herbal remedies for everyday aches and pains yields more positive results in that it's 100% natural, there are next to no side effects and they're rooted in our history. Almost every locality had their own herbal remedies for afflictions which consisted of ingredients that could be found around that locality or purchased from merchants.

The best part about many of the herbal remedies that you'll find is that they're all tried and tested and they can be easily made at home as well. The recipes contained within this eBook help relieve basic ailments and are easy to make as well as store.

However, do make sure that you're well aware of your medical condition before you start taking any of these herbal remedies. Furthermore, make sure to consult with your doctor or physician to make sure that you can safely follow these procedures. Used in moderation, these remedies can be an excellent alternative to popping pills all day.

Pharmaceutical medications have started to be frowned upon owing to the fact that their side effects are numerous and it is possible for one to develop any unhealthy addiction to such a drug. However, for people who're being ailed with aches and pains that require large doses of medication, herbal remedies can prove to be a God-sent alternative.

Herbal Recipes

Take a look at the following recipes and see which ones are suited to your condition or if you've tried them before or not.

Cleansing Cilantro Pesto

The seaweed in the recipe works with the herbs and gives it cleansing detox qualities.

Preparation time: 20 minutes

Ingredients

2 bunches of cilantro

1 bunch of arugula (can alternatively use dill, basil, parsley, rosemary, fennel, thyme, kale, etc.)

1 cup of sunflower seeds (raw, can alternatively use pumpkin seeds)

2 to 4 cloves of garlic

1 handful of toasted sea palm seaweed (can alternatively use toasted seaweed)

1 inch of ginger root (fresh, optional)

1 teaspoon of Miso (optional)

1 teaspoon sea salt (according to taste)

1 cup olive oil (can alternatively use sesame oil or hemp seed oil)

1 lime or lemon (juiced)

Method:

Finely chop herbs together and set them aside. Peel the ginger root and chop it finely as well. Use a food processor to blend the raw seeds, miso and garlic together. Make sure to add some olive oil to it. The oil should cover the ingredients. Blend for a few seconds on medium. Add the remaining olive oil, the lime juice and the chopped herbs to the mixture before covering and blending some more.

Continue blending on low speed and slowly bring the speed up to fast. Keep adding the olive oil to the mixture. Stop and scrape the ingredients down from the sides of the blender to make sure that all the ingredients mix well together.

Keep pulsing and adding olive oil until you get a mixture with a creamy, rich puree paste consistency. Store the mixture in jars and freeze or refrigerate.

Use:

Serve as is with vegetables, pasta, rice, meat dishes, etc. or any other savory dish.

Lemon Balm & Peppermint Infusion for Upset Stomachs

This soothing tea can be consumed throughout the day and helps sooth upset stomachs and menstrual pains while reducing stress and anxiety as well.

Preparation time: 20 minutes

Ingredients

2 teaspoon lemon balm leaves (dried)

2 teaspoon peppermint leaves (dried)

Lemon juice (according to taste, optional)

Honey (according to taste, optional)

Method:

Mix the dried leaves together and add them in one cup. Pour some boiling hot water to the mixture. Cover the cup with a lid and let the leaves steep for 10-20 minutes. Add some honey or lemon in it according to taste.

Use:

Have hot and drink no more than 2-3 cups per day.

Peppermint Foot-soak for Tired Feet

This foot soak helps treat tired muscles and sore feet as well as improving circulation. It's the perfect end-of-the-day foot soak to have after a tiring day. The foot soak is also soothing if you have cracks in your feet.

Preparation time: 20 minutes

Ingredients

½ cup peppermint leaves (dried)

or

1 cup peppermint leaves (fresh)

2 quarts of water

Method:

Prepare a foot bath by taking a large tub or a wash basin and layer it with the peppermint leaves. Take some water and allow it to boil on high heat. Pour the boiling water into the tub or wash basin and let the peppermint leaves steep in it for 10 minutes. Make sure all the leaves are submerged and soaked well.

Use:

Test the water before soaking your feet in it. If it is too hot for you, either wait a bit or add some cold water to cool it down. Soak feet in it for as long as you like.

Spearmint and Rosemary Tincture

Avoid consuming caffeine with the help of this herbal tincture. If you want to feel rejuvenated in mind or if you're working through the night and need something to keep your eyes open, give this tincture a try.

Preparation time: 2-6 weeks

Ingredients

1 cup rosemary leaves (fresh)

1 cup spearmint leave leaves (fresh)

1 bottle of Vodka (80 – 100 proof, unflavored, can use gin or brandy or even vinegar as well)

Method:

Finely chop the rosemary and spearmint leaves and set them aside in a large mason jar. Take the alcohol and pour it into the jar. Make sure that the chopped leaves are well immersed and covered with the mixture. If you're using vinegar, make sure to heat the vinegar slightly before pouring it into the jar.

Seal the jar carefully and tightly. Add a label to the container with the name and date on it. Store the jar at room temperature and make sure to give it a good shake after a few days.

Let the mixture rest for 2-6 weeks before you prepare to drain it. Take another jar and pour out the liquid into it. Use a cheese cloth over the mouth of the jar to pour out the mixture but hold back the herbs. Squeeze the cloth to make sure that all the liquid has been drained.

Use:

You can consume the tincture twice a day, every day. Make sure to mix one tablespoon with a glass of water.

Lavender and Chamomile Body Cream

This lovely, sweet smelling cream is particularly soothing for sun-burned skin and diaper rashes. You can also use it if you just love the smell of lavender and chamomile.

Ingredients:

For the oil

Preparation time: 10 days

1/3 cup chamomile flower petals (dried)

Olive oil (as needed)

For the Body Cream

Preparation time: 20 minutes

½ cup of cocoa butter

½ cup of coconut oil

1 teaspoon of lavender essential oil (as pure as possible)

Method:

For the oil:

The first thing you need is a chamomile infused oil. You can easily make this at home. Take the dried chamomile flower petals and place them in a jar. Cover the petals with olive oil and make sure that the oil covers them. Leave the petals to soak in the oil but check the jar after an hour or two. Add more olive oil if the petals have absorbed any.

Place a clean cloth over the mouth of the jar and place the jar in an area that receives a good amount of sunlight. Leave the jar for 10 days before straining the oil out of the jar. Throw away or compost the petals.

For the Body Cream

Take a small saucepan and on medium to low heat, melt the cocoa butter with the coconut oil and 1 cup of the chamomile infused oil. Once the ingredients are combined, pour them into a stainless steel bowl and allow them to cool in the freezer.

Make sure to whip the mixture with the help of an electric mixer. Every few minutes place the mixture back in the freezer but whip again after a few minutes. Slowly, increase the speed of the mixer and bring it up to high.

Once the mixture starts to thicken and become creamy, take some essential oil (pure lavender) and fold it as gently as possible into the mixture.

Spoon the finished mixture into jars or containers made of glass. Make sure they have air tight lids. Store in a refrigerator or in a cool place.

Use:

You can apply the body cream whenever you want. If it's too solid for application, leave it to thaw a bit at room temperature before applying.

Plantain Cream for Insect Stings and Bites

For insect bites, stings, itching and swelling, the anti-inflammatory qualities of the plantain make it the perfect thing to apply when dealing with these conditions.

Preparation time: 40 minutes

Ingredients:

4 tablespoons of plantain leaves (fresh)

2/3 cups of water (boiling)

2 tablespoons of olive oil (can use sunflower oil instead)

2 tablespoons of almond oil

1 teaspoon of natural beeswax

2 teaspoons of emulsifying wax

2 teaspoons of glycerin

1 teaspoon of powdered Vitamin C

Method:

Make sure to chop and wash the plantain leaves before opting to use them. Divide them into bunches of two. Place one bunch in the pan and place the other plantain bunch in a bowl full of water. Leave them like that for 10 minutes in order to allow the plantain to infuse the water with its essence.

While the plantain is infusing in the water, add some olive oil to the plantain leaves in the pan and let them simmer gently on low heat. As soon as it simmers, remove from the heat and set it aside to cool down for 10 minutes. Do not let the oil come to a boil. Remove immediately from heat if that happens.

Drain the plantain leaves from the water infusion. Set the water aside in a different bowl. Similarly, take another pan and drain the plantain infused oil into it with the help of a strainer to get the plantain leaves out of it. Bring the oil up to heat again and then add the emulsifying wax and the beeswax to the mixture. Make sure to keep on stirring consistently until the waxes have melted. Keep stirring and make sure that the mixture is foamy in consistency.

Once you get that consistency, add a cup of the plantain infused water to the mixture in the pan. Keep a whisk in hand and whisk hard until the mixture has thickened in consistency and is more like a salad dressing. Add in the powdered Vitamin C and the glycerin.

Mix well and then pour the mixture into glass jars that have been sterilized before use. Store in a cool, dry place or you can also keep it refrigerated.

Use:

You can apply the plantain cream whenever you want. If it's too solid for application, leave it to thaw a bit at room temperature before applying it. Apply on the area that has been affected as frequently as required.

Chili Plasters for Muscle Aches

This works as a soothing treatment with deep-heat for sore and stiff muscles.

Preparation time: 30 minutes

Ingredients:

1 cup of chili peppers (Scotch Bonnet, orange)

4 tablespoons of mustard powder

1 cup of coconut oil (non fractionated)

6 teaspoons of beeswax

4 packets of dressing pads for wounds (gauze, 4 x 4 inches)

4 packets of wound dressings (adhesive, 4 x 4 inches)

Method:

Start by washing and slicing all the chili peppers as finely as possible. Take a large saucepan and combine the mustard powder, the coconut oil and the sliced peppers. Cover and heat the mixture gently for 2 minutes. Do not let it simmer or come to a boil. After the two minutes are up, turn the heat off and allow the mixture to cool in the saucepan and keep the lid of the saucepan on.

Once the mixture has cooled, take a sieve and place a piece of cheesecloth over it. Pour the cooled chili mixture through it and make sure to squeeze the oil out. Make sure that you have a bowl placed underneath the cheesecloth and sieve in order to collect the oil.

Once you've squeezed out all the oil from the chili cheese cloth. Take a sauce pan and pour the excreted oil into it. Bring the oil up to heat. As the oil heats up, add some beeswax to it and stir to allow the beeswax to dissolve. Make sure that the oil is at a gentle heat. Do not bring the mixture to a boil or simmer. After two minutes, remove the oil from the heat.

Take the gauze dressing pads and dip them well in the chili oil while it is hot. Make sure that they are saturated well. Once they're soaked, remove them and place them on wax paper to let them set. Once they're dry, you can put them in a plastic wrap and store them in the refrigerator.

Use:

To use, make sure to lay down an adhesive dressing before you place a pad on top of the affected area. Use a blanket to cover the pad and keep the area warm. Keep the chili pad on the affected for 30 minutes or 1 hour as often as required.

Note:

Do not substitute the chili with any other kind of chili for this recipe.

Licorice and Marshmallow Root Cough Syrup

For coughs and sore throats, this licorice and marshmallow root syrup can work wonders. It is especially great for dry, sore throats.

Preparation time: 30 minutes

Ingredients:

4 tablespoons of marshmallow root (dried, chopped roughly)

2 licorice roots (dried, roughly broken into smaller pieces)

3 bunches of elderberries (fresh)

1 teaspoon of cloves (well ground)

1 orange peel

1 teaspoon of anise (only seeds)

8 eucalyptus leaves (fresh)

2 cups of water

½ cup of honey

1 lime (juiced)

5 tablespoons of glycerin

Method:

Take a large pan and pour the cups of water into it. On low heat, add the licorice and marshmallow root, the elderberries, anise, orange peel, eucalyptus leaves and the cloves. Keep the heat low and let the mixture simmer slowly. Reduce the liquid in the pan almost by one-fifth. Make sure that the solution does not boil.

Once the solution has reduced, remove eucalyptus leaves and the licorice and discard it. Pour the mixture into a blender and blitz all the ingredients. Blend the mixture in a blender until smooth. Pour back into the pan and add the honey, lime juice, and glycerin, then stir and simmer for 2 minutes. Do not let the mixture come to a boil. Once the glycerin has dissolved, take off the heat and pour into glass jars that have been sterilized and are ready for use.

Use:

You can consume 2 tablespoons of this solution, 3 times a day to soothe your sore throat. Keep refrigerated.

Note:

Make sure to use within 2 weeks. If not completely consumed, discard the remaining solution and make a new batch for yourself since herbs in the solution will have lost their potency by that time.

If you intend to use fresh marshmallow root instead of dried marshmallow root, please make sure to add 8 tablespoons of marshmallow root and 4 tablespoons of dried licorice roots. The rest of the ingredients in the recipe will remain the same.

Calendula Balm for Blisters

This is a good, soothing balm for blisters and can be used for minor cuts and small abrasions as well.

Preparation time: 30 minutes

Ingredients:

2/3 cup of calendula oil

2 to 3 tablespoons of wax (emulsifying)

5 drops of essential oil (lavender)

5 drops of essential oil (tea tree)

Method:

Take a large pan and heat the calendula oil and the emulsifying wax together on low heat. Keep an eye on the wax and oil mix. Stir gently to make sure that the oil and wax are mixed well. Make sure that the wax has melted completely but it has not started to boil or simmer.

Remove from the heat and allow the mixture to cool a bit before adding the lavender and tea tree essential oils. Pour out into glass jars or covered tin cans for storage before the wax solidifies.

Use:

Use anytime, as required, after having cleaned the area. This is not a good balm for deep cuts or abrasions, so seek medical attention in any case where you may require stitches.

Anti-allergy Honey and Cinnamon Tea

Honey and Cinnamon have hypoallergenic qualities and can help ease, if not completely, soothe away your discomfort towards an allergic reaction such as hay fever.

Preparation time: 35 minutes

Ingredients:

1 to 2 sticks of Cinnamon

1 to 2 tablespoons of raw honey (organic)

Method:

Take 2 cups of water and bring them to a boil. Lower the heat and add the stick of cinnamon into it. Let it simmer slightly for 30 minutes or until the water starts to darken and you can smell the cinnamon essence.

Remove the cinnamon stick and pour out the cinnamon tea in a cup. Add a spoonful of raw honey and stir well.

If you want a stronger cinnamon taste, use 2 cinnamon sticks and 2 tablespoons of raw honey. If you do not have cinnamon bark sticks at home, use one teaspoon of cinnamon powder instead.

Use:

Use twice a day, to soothe symptoms that cause coughing, sneezing, wheezing, etc. Do not use it when dealing with peanut allergies as that requires immediate medical attention.

Soothing Rosemary Infused Herbal Bath Soak

This bath soak is great for arthritis pain, sore muscles, to reduce stress and for fibromyalgia. This bath is also great for use as a detoxifying agent.

Preparation time: 10 minutes

Ingredients:

2 cups of salts (Epsom or any other brand)

1 cup of bi-carbonate soda

10 drops of essential oil (peppermint)

5 drops essential oil (eucalyptus)

5 drops essential oil (rosemary)

5 drops essential oil (lavender)

5 drops essential oil (cinnamon)

2 tablespoons of flowers (dried, lavender)

1 tablespoon of rosemary leaves (fresh)

2 sprigs of rosemary (optional)

Method:

Take a large bowl and mix the bath salts and the bi-carbonated soda together. Slowly add all the essential oils and make sure to mix gently but well enough to make sure that all the oils are evenly mixed in with the salts.

Take the dried lavender flowers and rosemary leaves and crush them a bit to make them easier to stir into the bath salts. Put two rosemary sprigs into a glass jar with a lid and add the bath salt mixture into it. Close the lid and give the jar a good shake to make sure everything is mixed well.

If you don't have bath salts, you can make a strong rosemary and lavender tea using the lavender flowers and rosemary leaves. Don't add any bi-carbonated soda in this. Strain the leaves and flowers out of the tea and add all the essential oils in it before storing it in a glass jar.

Use:

Use 1 cup of the rosemary infused bath salts or ½ cup of the rosemary tea per bath. Make sure that the water is warm and soak for 10 to 15 minutes.

Use as frequently as needed.

Sore Muscle Balm

The anti-inflammatory and soothing qualities of this balm make it great for sore or aching muscles owing to fibromyalgia or every day wear and tear.

Preparation time: 20 minutes

Ingredients:

3 tablespoons of wax (emulsifying)

2/3 cup of olive oil

2 drops of essential oil (clove)

6 drops essential oil (eucalyptus)

4 drops essential oil (thyme)

Method:

Take a large pan and heat the olive oil and the emulsifying wax together on low heat. Keep an eye on the wax and oil mix. Stir gently to make sure that the oil and wax are mixed well. Make sure that the wax has melted completely but it has not started to boil or simmer.

Remove from the heat and allow the mixture to cool a bit before adding the clove, eucalyptus and thyme essential oils. Pour out into glass jars or covered tin cans for storage before the wax solidifies.

Use:

Use anytime, as required. For topical use only.

Herbal Essential Oil Blend for Headaches and Sinuses

The essential oils used in this blend complement each other and work to help counteract heavy headaches, colds, stuffy noses, and congestion and sinus headaches.

Preparation time: 10 minutes

Ingredients:

6 drops of essential oil (Rosemary)

4 drops essential oil (Pine)

4 drops essential oil (Eucalyptus)

2 drops of essential oil (Peppermint)

Method:

Simply mix all the oils together. Put the mixed oil blend in a glass jar and remember to label it along with the various oils used so that you do not forget what is in it.

Use:

For headaches, make a warm bath soak or a foot soak using the essential oil blend you created. Soak in it for 20 minutes to ease the head ache. You can also use an aroma lamp to clear the air around your surroundings by burning this essential oil diffusion. You can also use this same blend to help with sore muscles.

Triple Whammy Herbal Oil for Nausea

With three essential oils and three techniques to try at the same time, this herbal remedy curbs sinus headaches and nausea and helps you feel better sooner.

Preparation time: 10 minutes

Ingredients:

1 to 2 tablespoons of dried peppermint

1 teaspoon of raw honey

1 teaspoon of lemon juice

10 drops of essential oil (peppermint)

3 drops essential oil (Lemon)

1 tablespoon of olive oil

Method:

The Tea:

Brew a peppermint tea with the help of the dried peppermint. Put the dried peppermint in a cup and pour boiling hot water. Cover and set aside for 30 minutes in order to allow the peppermint to infuse the tea properly. Add the honey and lemon juice to the tea.

The Bath:

Prepare a warm bath and add 8 drops of the peppermint essential oil to the water as well as 2 drops of the lemon essential oil. You can also opt to tie some fresh peppermint leaves with one lemon wedge in a muslin bag and put it in the bath.

The Massage Oil:

Use 2 drops of the peppermint essential oil, 1 drop of the lemon essential oil and 1 tablespoon of olive oil to create some massage oil.

Use:

Drink the peppermint and lemon tea while soaking in the peppermint bath. Soak in the bath for 20 minutes. Once the bath is done, take the massage oil and gently massage your forehead, temples and your neck with it. Make sure to avoid the eye area.

Anti-depressant Lemon Balm Tea

Great as an anti-depressant, lemon balm tea is also good for winters since it increases body heat and is sweat-inducing. Peppermint on the other hand is a great mental stimulant and will help lift your mood.

Preparation time: 10 minutes

Ingredients:

1 to 2 tablespoons of dried lemon balm leaves (can use fresh as well)

1 teaspoon of peppermint leaves (dried or fresh)

1 teaspoon of Stevia leaves

Method:

Brew a peppermint tea with the help of the dried lemon balm and peppermint leaves. Put the dried lemon balm, stevia leaves and peppermint in a cup or a kettle and pour boiling hot water. Cover and set aside for 30 minutes in order to allow the herbs to infuse the tea properly.

Use:

Drink the peppermint and lemon balm tea while sitting in a calming environment. For added effect, heat some lavender oil on an aroma lamp and let the lavender smell and lemon balm tea sooth you.

Avena (Oats) Tincture for Nerve Pain

Avena or oats as they are commonly known are great at soothing jangled nerves. Its mild nature allows it to be utilized for anti-depression and to ease anxiety as well.

Preparation time: 2-6 weeks

Ingredients

1 teaspoon skullcap leaves (dried or fresh)

1 teaspoon St. John's Wort flowers (dried or fresh)

1 teaspoon of oats (fresh)

1 teaspoon of licorice root

½ a dropper of ginger essence

½ a dropper of vervian leaves

1 bottle of Vodka (80 – 100 proof, unflavored, can use gin or brandy or even vinegar as well)

Method:

Finely chop the herbs or mash the oats and set them aside in a large Mason jar. Take the alcohol and pour it into the Mason jar. Make sure that the chopped herbs and oats are well immersed and covered with the mixture. If you're using vinegar, make sure to heat the vinegar slightly before pouring it into the jar.

Seal the jar carefully and tightly. Add a label to the container with the name and date on it. Store the jar at room temperature and make sure to give it a good shake after a few dayso.

Let the mixture rest for 2-6 weeks before you prepare to drain it. Take another jar and pour out the liquid into it. Use a cheese cloth over the mouth of the jar to pour out the mixture but hold back the solids. Squeeze the cloth to make sure that all the liquid has been drained.

Use:

You can consume the tincture twice a day, every day. Make sure to mix one tablespoon with water, juices, teas or any other drink.

Anti-Fungal Sage Powder

This anti-fungal powder not only helps treat rashes and athlete's foot, it's also sweet smelling with sage and rosemary in it.

Preparation time: 20 minutes

Ingredients

1 cup dusting powder

1 tablespoon talcum powder (scentless)

1 tablespoon cornstarch powder

¼ cup baking soda

1 tablespoon of sage (fresh, well ground)

1 tablespoon of rosemary (fresh, well ground)

1 drop of essential oil (sage)

1 drop of essential oil (rosemary)

Method:

To start off, make a base powder with the help of the dusting powder. Take a small bowl and mix the dusting powder, the cornstarch, baking soda and the scentless talcum powder together.

Add the crushed herbs to the   +powder mixture and mix well to make sure that they're infused properly with the powder. Pour the powder into a glass jar and add the rosemary and sage essential oils to the powder. Close the lid and give it a good shake to make sure that the powder is mixed well.

Use:

You can opt to take an old talcum powder bottle and fill it with this herbal powder. Shake a small dusting on to the rash or fungal area. This powder is good with superficial fungal infections and is meant for topical use only. Consult a doctor if the infection is serious.

Anti-Chest Congestion Salve

Chest congestion can be a painful condition which often requires antibiotic medication to make it heal. This salve can help soothe the pain and discomfort that might accompany that condition.

Preparation time: 20 minutes

Ingredients

2/3 cup olive oil

3 tablespoons of wax (emulsifying)

2 tablespoons of camphor

3 tablespoons of powdered rosin

2 teaspoons of linseed oil (raw)

½ teaspoon of turpentine

Method:

Take a large pan and heat the olive oil and the emulsifying wax together on low heat. Keep an eye on the wax and oil mix. Stir gently to make sure that the oil and wax are mixed well. Make sure that the wax has melted completely but it has not started to boil or simmer.

Remove from the heat and allow the mixture to cool a bit before adding the camphor, rosin, turpentine and linseed oil. Pour out into glass jars or covered tin cans for storage before the wax solidifies.

Use:

Use as required. If condition worsens, seek medical attention immediately.

Elderberry Tincture for Flu

The elderberry helps soothe flu symptoms such as body aches and prevents the onset of fever while allowing the body to heal.

Preparation time: 2-6 weeks

Ingredients

½ cup of Elderberries (mashed)

8 cups of water

½ cup of honey (raw, organic)

1 bottle of Vodka (80 – 100 proof, unflavored, can use gin or brandy or even vinegar as well)

Method:

Boil the berries in the water. Turn the heat down to low and let the berries simmer until the liquid has been reduced down to 2 cups remaining. Pour into a mason jar. Add the vodka and the honey to the mixture.

Seal the jar carefully and tightly. Add a label to the container with the name and date on it. Store the jar at room temperature and make sure to give it a good shake after a few days.

Let the mixture rest for 2-6 weeks before you prepare to drain it. Take another jar and pour out the liquid into it. Use a cheese cloth over the mouth of the jar to pour out the mixture but hold back the solids. Squeeze the cloth to make sure that all the liquid has been drained.

Use:

You can consume the tincture twice a day, every day. Make sure to mix one tablespoon with water, juices, teas or any other drink.

Aloe Hand Sanitizer

Aloe is a natural cleanser and this all natural hand sanitizer with lavender and tea tree will not only keep your skin clean but fragrant and moisturized as well.

Preparation time: 20 minutes

Ingredients

1 cup of Aloe Vera gel (can harvest directly from the Aloe Vera plant)

1 teaspoon of rubbing alcohol

2 teaspoons of vegetable glycerin

5 drops essential oil (lavender)

5 drops of essential oil (tea tree)

Method:

Take a large bowl and mix the Aloe Vera gel, the glycerin and the rubbing alcohol. Mix well until all the components are completely combined. Add the essential oils and mix well again.

Store the finished sanitizer in an empty hand pump or in a jar.

Use:

As required. Do not consume since it is meant for external use only.

Good Night Sleep Remedy

Stress and anxiety can often trigger insomnia which can further increase the stress and anxiety you feel. Break the chain with the help of this sleep remedy.

Preparation time: 30 minutes

Ingredients

2 cups of hops (dried)

1 cup of chamomile flowers (dried)

1 cup of lavender flowers (dried)

3 drops of essential oil (lavender)

1 foot of Muslin fabric (or any other fabric)

Method:

Take a bowl and mix all the hops, chamomile flowers, lavender flowers with the essential oils.

Fold the fabric and cut a square of 8x8 inches. Start sewing the edges together and to close the square. Sew all three sides, leaving one side open like a pocket. Start filling the pocket with the herb mixture you prepared. Make sure to fill it completely with the herbs then sew the pocket shut.

Use:

Sleep with this herbal pillow near your head. The lavender, chamomile and hops will relax your mind allowing you to sleep peacefully and fitfully.

This remedy is only meant for moderate problems in sleeping. For more serious conditions, please consult a medical expert.

Nettle Beer for Joint Pain

Nettle has always been utilized for arthritic pains. In this delicious beverage, you'll be able to relieve your joint pains without enduring the bitter taste of nettles.

Preparation time: 16 days

Ingredients

1 pound of sugar (raw)

2 lemons

1 ounce of cream of tartar

5 liters of water

2 pounds of stinging nettle leaves (fresh)

1 ounce of yeast (live)

Method:

Take a bowl and start removing the lemon zest. Make sure there is no white in it. Juice the lemons in the bowl once their zest has been completely removed. Add the sugar and the cream of tartar in a crock pot and set aside.

Take a large pot and add the water to it. Allow it come to a boil then add the nettles in it. Lower the heat and let the nettles cook in it for almost 15 minutes before taking it off the heat.

Place a strainer over the crock and drain the nettle infused water into it and stir to let the sugar dissolve. Allow the water to cool in the crock. Take a small bowl and dissolve the yeast with the help of some water. Keep an eye on the nettle mixture's temperature in the crock though. As soon as the liquid reaches blood warm add the yeast to it and close the crock.

Take a large cloth and cover the crock in several folds of it. Let this mixture brew for four days. Finally open the crock and using a muslin cloth or a strainer, get all the solids and sediment out. Store the mixture in glass bottles or jars that have tight lids and be sure to label the date and ingredients. Shake the bottle every two days or so. After twelve days, the nettle beer will be ready.

Use:

Drink chilled or according to your own preference. For serious aches and pains, make sure to consult a physician before opting to treat it with nettle beer.

Rosemary Tea for Mental Focus

Rosemary acts as a mental stimulant and energizes the mind, It also helps to fight against depression and anxiety.

Preparation time: 15 minutes

Ingredients:

1 to 2 tablespoons of rosemary leaves (can use fresh as well)

1 teaspoon of raw honey (organic)

Method:

Brew a rosemary tea with the help of rosemary leaves. Put the dried rosemary leaves in a cup or a kettle and pour boiling hot water. Cover and set aside for 30 minutes in order to allow the herbs to infuse the tea properly.

Add the raw honey and stir well before drinking the rosemary tea.

Use:

Drink the rosemary tea twice a day and as often as required.

Herbal Body Wrap

This body wrap produces therapeutic benefits and even aids in cleansing the body, freeing it of toxins. It's also great for people who might suffer from inflammation and joint pain.

Preparation time: 20 minutes

Ingredients:

2 cups green clay, Dead Sea clay or bentonite

¼ cup of sea salt

½ cup of chamomile (powdered)

½ cup of parsley (powdered)

1 cup kelp (powdered)

2 drops of essential oil (lavender)

2 drops of essential oil (eucalyptus)

2 tablespoons of aloe vera (gel)

2 tablespoons of shea oil

1.8 liters water

Method:

Take a large pot and let the water come to a boil. Add the sea salt to it and let it dissolve in it completely. Once the sea salt has dissolved, add the shea oil, essential oils, powdered herbs, the aloe vera gel and the green clay and let them all dissolve as well.

Lower the heat and allow the mixture to reduce and thicken until it has a mud like consistency. Take off the heat and allow the herbal mud wrap to come down to blood temperature before using it.

Use:

Whenever needed. Apply the herbal body wrap generously on your body. Once you're covered in it, take a sheet or some cling wrap and wrap yourself as tightly as possible. You might want to ask someone to help cocoon you snugly.

Stay wrapped for an hour before taking off the cling wrap. Soak in a lavender infused bath to get the herbal body mud off.

Cayenne Pepper and Menthol Herbal Salve for Arthritis

While this herbal salve can bring immense relief and improve circulation from pain, it should be used with caution since it contains cayenne pepper. Cayenne can irritate skin so it is advisable to perform a skin test on a small area before applying it anywhere.

Preparation time: 20 days

Ingredients:

1 cup coconut oil

4 tablespoons of cayenne (powdered)

4 tablespoons of wax (emulsifying)

2 tablespoons of menthol crystals

10 drops of the essential oil (cinnamon)

10 drops of the essential oil (thuja)

10 drops of the essential oil (benzoin resin)

Method:

Heat the coconut oil and add the powdered cayenne to it. Mix well and put in a jar. Place the jar in a warm location such as a warm cupboard or a sunny window pane or anywhere else where you'll also be able to keep stirring it occasionally.

After 7 – 10 days, stop stirring the mixture and let it rest completely. Allow the powder to settle to the bottom of the jar. This may take another 2-3 days before the oil starts to clear. Once the oil is clearer, open the jar and remove the clean oil from the top. Throw away the oil with the residue and gunk in it.

Take the emulsifying wax and melt it in the microwave or on the stove on low heat. Heat the clarified cayenne-coconut oil and mix it in with the melted wax. Do not let the wax simmer or boil.

Add the menthol crystals and stir until they are completely dissolved. Add in the essential oils and stir until they are all mixed well. Pour into a jar and store in a cool dry space. Refrigerate if needed when days are too warm and the salve becomes too runny.

Use:

Apply on the area where the body is aching. You can also apply this salve to improve blood circulation and relieve nerve pain in certain areas of the body. Be sure to consult a physician and conduct a skin patch test before using this salve.